LiveReal
JOURNAL

A MEDICAL PLANNER TO
HELP WITH APPOINTMENTS,
MEDICATIONS, AND CARETAKING

by
SAMANTHA MELANEY

GLOBAL WELLNESS MEDIA
STRATEGIC EDGE INNOVATIONS PUBLISHING
LOS ANGELES, TORONTO, MONTREAL

For permission requests, send an email to
book@samanthamelaney.com

First Edition. Published by:
Global Wellness Media
Strategic Edge Innovations Publishing
440 N Barranca Ave #2027
Covina, California 91723-1722
(866) 467-9090
StrategicEdgeInnovations.com

Book Design: Global Wellness Media
Cover Design: Eric D. Groleau

LiveReal Journal/ Samantha Melaney. — 1st ed.
ISBN: 978- (Paperback)

"God helps us become stronger than the storm, whatever the type of storm it may be."

—Samantha Melaney

TABLE OF CONTENTS

INTRODUCTION

INTRODUCTION

Hello my friend!

I want to briefly explain how this special journal came to be. For years when I was caring for my daughter who has a liver disease, I carried a small notebook to every appointment where I would record everything that was said and done, good and bad. I also noted what needed to be done for her on the days between her appointments. I tracked everything regarding her care.

Although my little notebook was helpful, I have designed this one to be what I wish I would have had then. Whether you are caring for someone you love or yourself, I believe this journal will help you.

With Love,

Samantha Melaney

Author & Liver Momma

For more information, check out the video about this journal at

samanthamelaney.com

AFFIRMATIONS

I believe affirmations are powerful. Here are a few that I love that you can use to get started. Feel free to change them and add your own..

I AM STRONG
I AM LOVED
I AM GRATEFUL
I LOOK FOR WHAT I CAN LEARN
I LOOK FOR WAYS TO HELP OTHERS

MY OWN AFFIRMATIONS:

PAST CHALLENGES

Past challenges prepare us for future ones...

What hard experiences have I already survived?

I know it may not seem the same. It might feel a lot smaller than what you are going through now, but reflecting on past challenges can help give you strength for your current challenge(s).

HARD THINGS I'VE BEEN THROUGH:

CONTACTS & INFORMATION

CONTACTS & INFORMATION

CONTACTS & INFORMATION

CONTACTS & INFORMATION

CONTACTS & INFORMATION

CONTACTS & INFORMATION

CONTACTS & INFORMATION

CALENDAR

CALENDAR

Month ____________________

SUNDAY	MONDAY	TUESDAY	WEDNESDAY	THURSDAY	FRIDAY	SATURDAY

Notes

____

____

____

CALENDAR

Month ____________________

SUNDAY	MONDAY	TUESDAY	WEDNESDAY	THURSDAY	FRIDAY	SATURDAY

Notes

____

____

____

CALENDAR

Month ____________________

SUNDAY	MONDAY	TUESDAY	WEDNESDAY	THURSDAY	FRIDAY	SATURDAY

Notes

____

____

____

CALENDAR

Month ____________________

SUNDAY	MONDAY	TUESDAY	WEDNESDAY	THURSDAY	FRIDAY	SATURDAY

Notes

____

____

____

CALENDAR

Month ____________________

SUNDAY	MONDAY	TUESDAY	WEDNESDAY	THURSDAY	FRIDAY	SATURDAY

Notes

____

____

____

CALENDAR

Month ________________

SUNDAY	MONDAY	TUESDAY	WEDNESDAY	THURSDAY	FRIDAY	SATURDAY

Notes

____

____

____

CALENDAR

Month ____________________

SUNDAY	MONDAY	TUESDAY	WEDNESDAY	THURSDAY	FRIDAY	SATURDAY

Notes

____

____

____

CALENDAR

Month ____________________

SUNDAY	MONDAY	TUESDAY	WEDNESDAY	THURSDAY	FRIDAY	SATURDAY

Notes

____

____

____

CALENDAR

Month ____________________

SUNDAY	MONDAY	TUESDAY	WEDNESDAY	THURSDAY	FRIDAY	SATURDAY

Notes

____

____

____

CALENDAR

Month ____________________

SUNDAY	MONDAY	TUESDAY	WEDNESDAY	THURSDAY	FRIDAY	SATURDAY

Notes

___

___

___

CALENDAR

Month ____________________

SUNDAY	MONDAY	TUESDAY	WEDNESDAY	THURSDAY	FRIDAY	SATURDAY

Notes

____

____

____

CALENDAR

Month ____________________

SUNDAY	MONDAY	TUESDAY	WEDNESDAY	THURSDAY	FRIDAY	SATURDAY

Notes

____

____

____

APPOINTMENTS

APPOINTMENT

Date ______________________ Weight ______________________

Doctor ______________________ Height ______________________

Lab Results

Questions / Discussions / Notes

Medication Changes

Next Appointment Date ______________________

APPOINTMENT

Date ____________________ Weight ____________________

Doctor ____________________ Height ____________________

Lab Results

Questions / Discussions / Notes

Medication Changes

Next Appointment Date ____________________

APPOINTMENT

Date ____________________ Weight ____________________

Doctor ____________________ Height ____________________

Lab Results

Questions / Discussions / Notes

Medication Changes

Next Appointment Date ____________________

APPOINTMENT

Date ____________________ Weight ____________________

Doctor ____________________ Height ____________________

Lab Results

Questions / Discussions / Notes

Medication Changes

Next Appointment Date ____________________

APPOINTMENT

Date ______________________ Weight ______________________

Doctor ______________________ Height ______________________

Lab Results

Questions / Discussions / Notes

Medication Changes

Next Appointment Date ______________________

APPOINTMENT

Date ____________________ Weight ____________________

Doctor ____________________ Height ____________________

Lab Results

Questions / Discussions / Notes

Medication Changes

Next Appointment Date ____________________

APPOINTMENT

Date ____________________ Weight ____________________

Doctor ____________________ Height ____________________

Lab Results

Questions / Discussions / Notes

Medication Changes

Next Appointment Date ____________________

APPOINTMENT

Date ______________________ Weight ____________________

Doctor ______________________ Height ____________________

Lab Results

____

____

____

____

Questions / Discussions / Notes

____

____

____

____

____

____

____

____

Medication Changes

____

____

____

____

____

Next Appointment Date ______________________________

APPOINTMENT

Date ______________________ Weight ______________________

Doctor ______________________ Height ______________________

Lab Results

Questions / Discussions / Notes

Medication Changes

Next Appointment Date ______________________

APPOINTMENT

Date ______________________ Weight ______________________

Doctor ______________________ Height ______________________

Lab Results

Questions / Discussions / Notes

Medication Changes

Next Appointment Date ______________________

APPOINTMENT

Date ______________________ Weight ______________________

Doctor ______________________ Height ______________________

Lab Results

____

____

____

____

Questions / Discussions / Notes

____

____

____

____

____

____

____

____

Medication Changes

____

____

____

____

____

Next Appointment Date ______________________

APPOINTMENT

Date ______________________ Weight ____________________

Doctor ______________________ Height ____________________

Lab Results

Questions / Discussions / Notes

Medication Changes

Next Appointment Date ______________________

APPOINTMENT

Date ____________________ Weight ____________________

Doctor ____________________ Height ____________________

Lab Results

Questions / Discussions / Notes

Medication Changes

Next Appointment Date ____________________

APPOINTMENT

Date ____________________ Weight ____________________

Doctor ____________________ Height ____________________

Lab Results

Questions / Discussions / Notes

Medication Changes

Next Appointment Date ____________________

APPOINTMENT

Date ______________________ Weight ______________________

Doctor ______________________ Height ______________________

Lab Results

Questions / Discussions / Notes

Medication Changes

Next Appointment Date ______________________

APPOINTMENT

Date ____________________ Weight ____________________

Doctor ____________________ Height ____________________

Lab Results

Questions / Discussions / Notes

Medication Changes

Next Appointment Date ____________________

APPOINTMENT

Date ______________________ Weight ______________________

Doctor ______________________ Height ______________________

Lab Results

____

____

____

____

Questions / Discussions / Notes

____

____

____

____

____

____

____

____

Medication Changes

____

____

____

____

____

Next Appointment Date ______________________

APPOINTMENT

Date ______________________ Weight ______________________

Doctor ______________________ Height ______________________

Lab Results

Questions / Discussions / Notes

Medication Changes

Next Appointment Date ______________________

APPOINTMENT

Date ______________________ Weight ______________________

Doctor ______________________ Height ______________________

Lab Results

____

____

____

____

Questions / Discussions / Notes

____

____

____

____

____

____

____

____

Medication Changes

____

____

____

____

____

Next Appointment Date ______________________

APPOINTMENT

Date ______________________ Weight ______________________

Doctor ______________________ Height ______________________

Lab Results

____

____

____

____

Questions / Discussions / Notes

____

____

____

____

____

____

____

____

Medication Changes

____

____

____

____

____

Next Appointment Date ______________________

APPOINTMENT

Date ____________________ Weight ____________________

Doctor ____________________ Height ____________________

Lab Results

Questions / Discussions / Notes

Medication Changes

Next Appointment Date ____________________

APPOINTMENT

Date ____________________ Weight ____________________

Doctor ____________________ Height ____________________

Lab Results

Questions / Discussions / Notes

Medication Changes

Next Appointment Date ____________________

APPOINTMENT

Date ______________________ Weight ______________________

Doctor ______________________ Height ______________________

Lab Results

Questions / Discussions / Notes

Medication Changes

Next Appointment Date ______________________

APPOINTMENT

Date ______________________ Weight ______________________

Doctor ______________________ Height ______________________

Lab Results

____

____

____

____

Questions / Discussions / Notes

____

____

____

____

____

____

____

____

Medication Changes

____

____

____

____

____

Next Appointment Date ______________________

APPOINTMENT

Date ______________________ Weight ______________________

Doctor ______________________ Height ______________________

Lab Results

____

____

____

____

Questions / Discussions / Notes

____

____

____

____

____

____

____

____

Medication Changes

____

____

____

____

____

Next Appointment Date ______________________

APPOINTMENT

Date ____________________ Weight ____________________

Doctor ____________________ Height ____________________

Lab Results

Questions / Discussions / Notes

Medication Changes

Next Appointment Date ____________________

MEDICATIONS

MEDICATIONS

Date ______________________

Fridge	Medication / Dose / Frequency	AM	PM
Y/N		☐	☐
Y/N		☐	☐
Y/N		☐	☐
Y/N		☐	☐
Y/N		☐	☐
Y/N		☐	☐
Y/N		☐	☐
Y/N		☐	☐
Y/N		☐	☐
Y/N		☐	☐
Y/N		☐	☐
Y/N		☐	☐
Y/N		☐	☐
Y/N		☐	☐
Y/N		☐	☐

Notes of Symptoms / Side Effects

MEDICATIONS

Date ___________________

Fridge	Medication / Dose / Frequency	AM	PM
Y / N		☐	☐
Y / N		☐	☐
Y / N		☐	☐
Y / N		☐	☐
Y / N		☐	☐
Y / N		☐	☐
Y / N		☐	☐
Y / N		☐	☐
Y / N		☐	☐
Y / N		☐	☐
Y / N		☐	☐
Y / N		☐	☐
Y / N		☐	☐
Y / N		☐	☐
Y / N		☐	☐

Notes of Symptoms / Side Effects

MEDICATIONS

Date ____________________

Fridge	Medication / Dose / Frequency	AM	PM
Y / N		☐	☐
Y / N		☐	☐
Y / N		☐	☐
Y / N		☐	☐
Y / N		☐	☐
Y / N		☐	☐
Y / N		☐	☐
Y / N		☐	☐
Y / N		☐	☐
Y / N		☐	☐
Y / N		☐	☐
Y / N		☐	☐
Y / N		☐	☐
Y / N		☐	☐
Y / N		☐	☐

Notes of Symptoms / Side Effects

MEDICATIONS

Date ______________________

Fridge	Medication / Dose / Frequency	AM	PM
Y / N		☐	☐
Y / N		☐	☐
Y / N		☐	☐
Y / N		☐	☐
Y / N		☐	☐
Y / N		☐	☐
Y / N		☐	☐
Y / N		☐	☐
Y / N		☐	☐
Y / N		☐	☐
Y / N		☐	☐
Y / N		☐	☐
Y / N		☐	☐
Y / N		☐	☐
Y / N		☐	☐

Notes of Symptoms / Side Effects

MEDICATIONS

Date ____________________

Fridge	Medication / Dose / Frequency	AM	PM
Y/N		☐	☐
Y/N		☐	☐
Y/N		☐	☐
Y/N		☐	☐
Y/N		☐	☐
Y/N		☐	☐
Y/N		☐	☐
Y/N		☐	☐
Y/N		☐	☐
Y/N		☐	☐
Y/N		☐	☐
Y/N		☐	☐
Y/N		☐	☐
Y/N		☐	☐
Y/N		☐	☐

Notes of Symptoms / Side Effects

MEDICATIONS

Date ______________________

Fridge	Medication / Dose / Frequency	AM	PM
Y / N		☐	☐
Y / N		☐	☐
Y / N		☐	☐
Y / N		☐	☐
Y / N		☐	☐
Y / N		☐	☐
Y / N		☐	☐
Y / N		☐	☐
Y / N		☐	☐
Y / N		☐	☐
Y / N		☐	☐
Y / N		☐	☐
Y / N		☐	☐
Y / N		☐	☐
Y / N		☐	☐

Notes of Symptoms / Side Effects

MEDICATIONS

Date ____________________

Fridge	Medication / Dose / Frequency	AM	PM
Y / N		☐	☐
Y / N		☐	☐
Y / N		☐	☐
Y / N		☐	☐
Y / N		☐	☐
Y / N		☐	☐
Y / N		☐	☐
Y / N		☐	☐
Y / N		☐	☐
Y / N		☐	☐
Y / N		☐	☐
Y / N		☐	☐
Y / N		☐	☐
Y / N		☐	☐
Y / N		☐	☐

Notes of Symptoms / Side Effects

MEDICATIONS

Date ______________________

Fridge	Medication / Dose / Frequency	AM	PM
Y / N		☐	☐
Y / N		☐	☐
Y / N		☐	☐
Y / N		☐	☐
Y / N		☐	☐
Y / N		☐	☐
Y / N		☐	☐
Y / N		☐	☐
Y / N		☐	☐
Y / N		☐	☐
Y / N		☐	☐
Y / N		☐	☐
Y / N		☐	☐
Y / N		☐	☐
Y / N		☐	☐

Notes of Symptoms / Side Effects

MEDICATIONS

Date ______________________

Fridge	Medication / Dose / Frequency	AM	PM
Y/N		☐	☐
Y/N		☐	☐
Y/N		☐	☐
Y/N		☐	☐
Y/N		☐	☐
Y/N		☐	☐
Y/N		☐	☐
Y/N		☐	☐
Y/N		☐	☐
Y/N		☐	☐
Y/N		☐	☐
Y/N		☐	☐
Y/N		☐	☐
Y/N		☐	☐
Y/N		☐	☐

Notes of Symptoms / Side Effects

MEDICATIONS

Date ____________________

Fridge	Medication / Dose / Frequency	AM	PM
Y / N		☐	☐
Y / N		☐	☐
Y / N		☐	☐
Y / N		☐	☐
Y / N		☐	☐
Y / N		☐	☐
Y / N		☐	☐
Y / N		☐	☐
Y / N		☐	☐
Y / N		☐	☐
Y / N		☐	☐
Y / N		☐	☐
Y / N		☐	☐
Y / N		☐	☐
Y / N		☐	☐

Notes of Symptoms / Side Effects

MEDICATIONS

Date ______________________

Fridge	Medication / Dose / Frequency	AM	PM
Y / N		☐	☐
Y / N		☐	☐
Y / N		☐	☐
Y / N		☐	☐
Y / N		☐	☐
Y / N		☐	☐
Y / N		☐	☐
Y / N		☐	☐
Y / N		☐	☐
Y / N		☐	☐
Y / N		☐	☐
Y / N		☐	☐
Y / N		☐	☐
Y / N		☐	☐
Y / N		☐	☐

Notes of Symptoms / Side Effects

MEDICATIONS

Date ______________________

Fridge	Medication / Dose / Frequency	AM	PM
Y / N		☐	☐
Y / N		☐	☐
Y / N		☐	☐
Y / N		☐	☐
Y / N		☐	☐
Y / N		☐	☐
Y / N		☐	☐
Y / N		☐	☐
Y / N		☐	☐
Y / N		☐	☐
Y / N		☐	☐
Y / N		☐	☐
Y / N		☐	☐
Y / N		☐	☐
Y / N		☐	☐

Notes of Symptoms / Side Effects

MEDICATIONS

Date ____________________

Fridge	Medication / Dose / Frequency	AM	PM
Y/N		☐	☐
Y/N		☐	☐
Y/N		☐	☐
Y/N		☐	☐
Y/N		☐	☐
Y/N		☐	☐
Y/N		☐	☐
Y/N		☐	☐
Y/N		☐	☐
Y/N		☐	☐
Y/N		☐	☐
Y/N		☐	☐
Y/N		☐	☐
Y/N		☐	☐
Y/N		☐	☐

Notes of Symptoms / Side Effects

MEDICATIONS

Date ______________________

Fridge	Medication / Dose / Frequency	AM	PM
Y / N		☐	☐
Y / N		☐	☐
Y / N		☐	☐
Y / N		☐	☐
Y / N		☐	☐
Y / N		☐	☐
Y / N		☐	☐
Y / N		☐	☐
Y / N		☐	☐
Y / N		☐	☐
Y / N		☐	☐
Y / N		☐	☐
Y / N		☐	☐
Y / N		☐	☐
Y / N		☐	☐

Notes of Symptoms / Side Effects

MEDICATIONS

Date ____________________

Fridge	Medication / Dose / Frequency	AM	PM
Y/N		☐	☐
Y/N		☐	☐
Y/N		☐	☐
Y/N		☐	☐
Y/N		☐	☐
Y/N		☐	☐
Y/N		☐	☐
Y/N		☐	☐
Y/N		☐	☐
Y/N		☐	☐
Y/N		☐	☐
Y/N		☐	☐
Y/N		☐	☐
Y/N		☐	☐
Y/N		☐	☐

Notes of Symptoms / Side Effects

MEDICATIONS

Date ______________________

Fridge	Medication / Dose / Frequency	AM	PM
Y / N		☐	☐
Y / N		☐	☐
Y / N		☐	☐
Y / N		☐	☐
Y / N		☐	☐
Y / N		☐	☐
Y / N		☐	☐
Y / N		☐	☐
Y / N		☐	☐
Y / N		☐	☐
Y / N		☐	☐
Y / N		☐	☐
Y / N		☐	☐
Y / N		☐	☐
Y / N		☐	☐

Notes of Symptoms / Side Effects

FOOD LOG

FOOD LOG

Date ____________________

Food / Fluids

Notes of Symptoms / Side Effects

FOOD LOG

Date

Food / Fluids

Notes of Symptoms / Side Effects

FOOD LOG

Date ______________________

Food / Fluids

Notes of Symptoms / Side Effects

FOOD LOG

Date ____________________

Food / Fluids

Notes of Symptoms / Side Effects

FOOD LOG

Date ______________________

Food / Fluids

Notes of Symptoms / Side Effects

FOOD LOG

Date ______________________

Food / Fluids

Notes of Symptoms / Side Effects

FOOD LOG

Date ______________________

Food / Fluids

Notes of Symptoms / Side Effects

FOOD LOG

Date ______________________

Food / Fluids

Notes of Symptoms / Side Effects

FOOD LOG

Date ______________________

Food / Fluids

Notes of Symptoms / Side Effects

FOOD LOG

Date ________________________

Food / Fluids

Notes of Symptoms / Side Effects

FOOD LOG

Date ____________________

Food / Fluids

Notes of Symptoms / Side Effects

FOOD LOG

Date ______________________

Food / Fluids

Notes of Symptoms / Side Effects

FOOD LOG

Date ______________________

Food / Fluids

Notes of Symptoms / Side Effects

FOOD LOG

Date ______________________

Food / Fluids

Notes of Symptoms / Side Effects

FOOD LOG

Date ____________________

Food / Fluids

Notes of Symptoms / Side Effects

FOOD LOG

Date ______________________

Food / Fluids

Notes of Symptoms / Side Effects

FOOD LOG

Date ____________________

Food / Fluids

Notes of Symptoms / Side Effects

FOOD LOG

Date ______________________

Food / Fluids

Notes of Symptoms / Side Effects

FOOD LOG

Date ______________________

Food / Fluids

Notes of Symptoms / Side Effects

FOOD LOG

Date ______________________

Food / Fluids

Notes of Symptoms / Side Effects

HOSPITAL JOURNAL

HOSPITAL JOURNAL

Date ____________________

Gratitude

____

____

____

____

____

Feeling

____

____

____

____

____

Win of the Day

____

____

____

____

____

HOSPITAL JOURNAL

Date ____________________

Gratitude

Feeling

Win of the Day

HOSPITAL JOURNAL

Date ______________________

Gratitude

____

____

____

____

____

Feeling

____

____

____

____

____

Win of the Day

____

____

____

____

____

HOSPITAL JOURNAL

Date ______________________

Gratitude

____

____

____

____

____

Feeling

____

____

____

____

____

Win of the Day

____

____

____

____

____

HOSPITAL JOURNAL

Date ______________________

Gratitude

Feeling

Win of the Day

HOSPITAL JOURNAL

Date ______________________

Gratitude

____

____

____

____

____

Feeling

____

____

____

____

____

Win of the Day

____

____

____

____

____

HOSPITAL JOURNAL

Date ____________________

Gratitude

Feeling

Win of the Day

HOSPITAL JOURNAL

Date ______________________

Gratitude

Feeling

Win of the Day

HOSPITAL JOURNAL

Date ____________________

Gratitude

Feeling

Win of the Day

HOSPITAL JOURNAL

Date ________________________

Gratitude

Feeling

Win of the Day

HOSPITAL JOURNAL

Date ______________________

Gratitude

____

____

____

____

____

Feeling

____

____

____

____

____

Win of the Day

____

____

____

____

____

HOSPITAL JOURNAL

Date ______________________

Gratitude

____

____

____

____

____

Feeling

____

____

____

____

____

Win of the Day

____

____

____

____

____

HOSPITAL JOURNAL

Date ____________________

Gratitude

Feeling

Win of the Day

HOSPITAL JOURNAL

Date ______________________

Gratitude

Feeling

Win of the Day

HOSPITAL JOURNAL

Date ______________________

Gratitude

Feeling

Win of the Day

HOSPITAL JOURNAL

Date

Gratitude

Feeling

Win of the Day

HOSPITAL JOURNAL

Date ____________________

Gratitude

Feeling

Win of the Day

HOSPITAL JOURNAL

Date ______________________

Gratitude

Feeling

Win of the Day

HOSPITAL JOURNAL

Date ______________________

Gratitude

Feeling

Win of the Day

HOSPITAL JOURNAL

Date ______________________

Gratitude

____

____

____

____

____

Feeling

____

____

____

____

____

Win of the Day

____

____

____

____

____

HOSPITAL JOURNAL

Date ____________________

Gratitude

Feeling

Win of the Day

HOSPITAL JOURNAL

Date ______________________

Gratitude

Feeling

Win of the Day

NOTES

NOTES

NOTES

NOTES

NOTES

LIVEREAL

FROM THE AUTHOR

The LiveReal Journal is intended for those who are caring for someone, whether it be a child, partner, parent, or themselves. It is meant to help keep track of appointments, medications, and other important details.

No matter the diagnosis this journal will assist in staying organized and up to date on caretaking needs.

Samantha Melaney

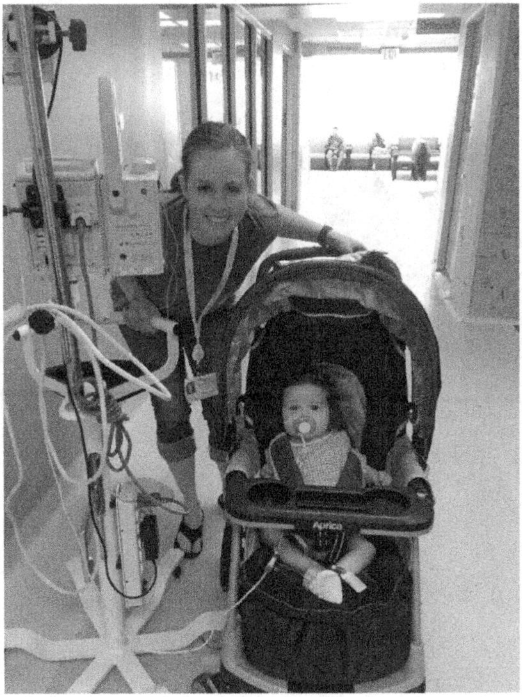

LIVEREAL

LiveReal recounts a family's journey through their daughter's liver transplant. It is a story of faith and miracles, following a life-threatening diagnosis of Biliary Atresia. This story provides a candid portrait of the fears, struggles, and hard decisions that her loving parents had to face. From a Kasai surgery to the prospect of a second transplant, the family experienced the beauty and heartache of life events.

A strong family bond with an unshakable faith made the dreadful wait for a transplant easier, yet the challenges of raising a young family while living part time in a hospital were significant.

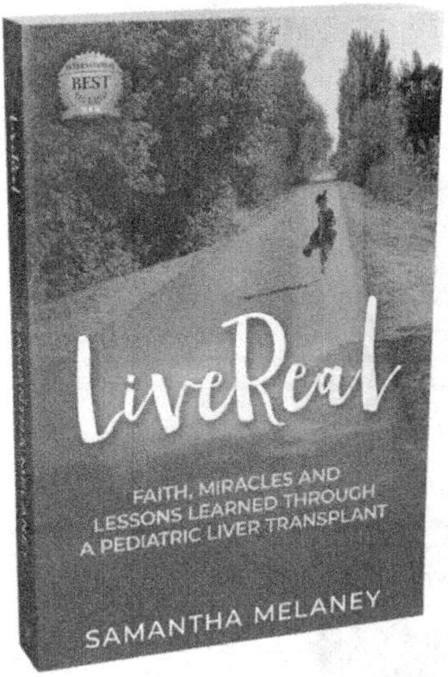

This book will provide hope and support to families that might be going through similar situations or inspire anyone dealing with challenges. It relates a powerful story and highlights important tips and lessons learned. Kendyl's pediatric journey will inspire you to keep going, and to face any obstacle with courage.

SAMANTHA MELANEY

SAMANTHA is passionate about living a life of purpose and encouraging others to do the same through physical, mental, and emotional growth.

As an author, speaker, and mentor, she uses the lessons learned from her family's journey to inspire people to keep their faith during hard times. She also raises awareness for organ donation by sharing her daughter's story of receiving a lifesaving pediatric liver transplant.

Samantha lives with her husband and two beautiful girls in Utah, USA.

For more information about Samantha and her family, please visit: https://SamanthaMelaney.com

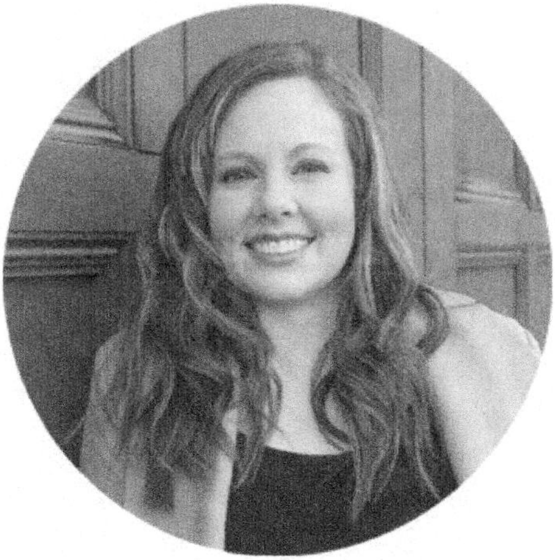

.

Made in the USA
Monee, IL
04 November 2026

67377413R00085